XYZ

Is the ABC of ECG

XYZ
Is the ABC of ECG

An Introduction to
QRS-T Interpretation for
Medical Students, Interns, Nurses
and ECG Technicians

IRWIN HOFFMAN, M.D.

*Associate Professor of Clinical Medicine, State University of
New York, Health Sciences Center, Stony Brook;
Attending Physician in Charge, ECG-VCG Laboratory,
Long Island Jewish-Hillside Medical Center;
Physician in Charge, ECG and VCG, South Nassau
Communities Hospital, Oceanside, New York*

YEAR BOOK MEDICAL PUBLISHERS · INC.
35 EAST WACKER DRIVE · CHICAGO

Library of Congress Catalog Card Number: 72-85705

International Standard Book Number: 0-8151-4542-X

To Maya, Minnie, Annabelle *and* John

Table of Contents

Introduction

Electrocardiographic interpretation is generally divided into two parts:

1. Analysis of cardiac rhythm and rhythm disorders.
2. Analysis of QRS-T complexes.

At the Long Island Jewish Medical Center, we have developed a simple and effective method for introducing the medical student, intern, nurse, or ECG technician to the subject of QRS and T interpretation. This brief handbook is devoted solely to an understanding of QRS-T complexes. We emphasize from the beginning that the material presented here cannot teach a student to interpret the ECG. The only way a student can become proficient in the interpretation of clinical electrocardiographic material is by studying and observing at the side of an expert electrocardiographer, preferably daily, for three to six months. Such daily exercises, combined with appropriate reading assignments, will lead the young physician to the point where he is able to take on the responsibility of interpreting electrocardiograms on his own.

This text was written to introduce the beginner to the general subject of QRS-T analysis, and, perhaps more important, to give him the information he needs to understand *an interpreted* ECG. The diagrams and illustrations are planned so that they may be easily projected or copied for use in teaching exercises.

What Is an Electrocardiogram?

Each cardiac contraction is associated with the production of a minute amount of electricity. This tiny voltage, measuring about 1/1000 of a volt (1 *milli*volt), may be amplified by appropriate equipment (the electrocardiograph machine) and then displayed in many different ways. In one form of display, the electrocardiogram, the fluctuations in this minute voltage during each heartbeat are recorded in permanent form on graph paper. A finished record might look like Figure 1.

Fig. 1.—A sample electrocardiogram (ECG), with *P, QRS,* and *T* waves occurring in an orderly sequence. The *QRS* wave (or "depolarization" wave) precedes mechanical cardiac contraction. The *T* wave represents recharging (or "repolarization") and thus prepares the heart for the next beat.

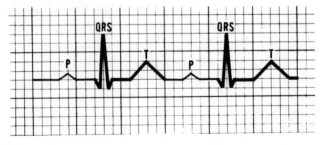

The QRS and T waves of the electrocardiogram occur in pairs during each successive heartbeat. The QRS is generally of higher voltage than the T. The QRS may be compared to

Fig. 2.—Various *QRS* complexes with positive or negative *T* waves.

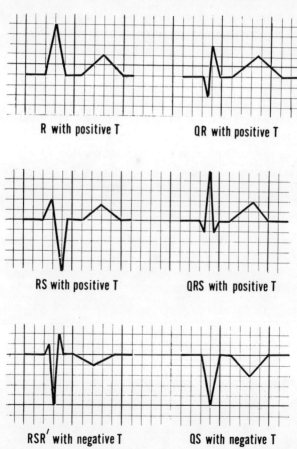

R with positive T   QR with positive T

RS with positive T   QRS with positive T

RSR' with negative T   QS with negative T

a fast battery discharge ("depolarization"), something like the discharge of a flashgun on a camera. The T, which is of lower amplitude but longer duration, may be likened to the recharging ("repolarization") of that battery in order to provide the next flash.

It is important to know the names of the various kinds of QRS complexes as they are encountered in electrocardiograms. An upright deflection from the baseline is called an R wave. A negative deflection is called an S wave. However, an *initial* negative deflection, if followed by a positive R wave, is called a Q wave. A positive-negative-positive sequence is called R-S-R'. (Figure 2 illustrates various kinds of QRS complexes.) T waves are easy to name. They are called positive if the wave is upright and negative if the wave is below the baseline. Observe the positive or negative T waves in each of the QRS-T complexes shown in Figure 2.

Time Intervals

The paper speed of most electrocardiograph machines is 25 millimeters (mm) per second. The graphic chart paper is ruled off in squares, 1 mm on a side. Thus, with the paper running at 25 mm per second, a 1-mm square corresponds to 1/25th of a second. This is usually written as 0.04 seconds, but may also be written as 40 milliseconds, or 40 msec.

Examine Figure 3 and measure the *duration* of the total QRS complex, of the Q wave alone, and of the *total* interval beginning with the Q and ending with the end of the T wave (Q-T interval).

The positive or negative QRS and T deflections have a *magnitude* measured in *millivolts* (1/1000 of a volt, abbreviated as "mv"). The electrocardiograph machine is

Fig. 3.—QRS duration = two time boxes, or 2 x 0.04 seconds, or 0.08 seconds. The duration of Q = one-half time box, or 0.04 seconds divided by 2, or 0.02 seconds. The duration of Q-T = eight time boxes or 8 x 0.04 seconds, or 0.32 seconds.

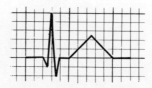

5

standardized by the technician so that a standard 1-mv impulse produces a deflection of 10 mm (10 *vertical* boxes in the finished record).

Examine Figure 4 and estimate the *amplitude* of the Q wave, the R wave, and the T wave. Note the standardizing impulse which has a magnitude of 1 mv.

Fig. 4.—Q amplitude = -2 voltage boxes, or -0.2 mv. R amplitude = +7 voltage boxes, or +0.7 mv. T amplitude = +4½ voltage boxes, or +0.45 mv.

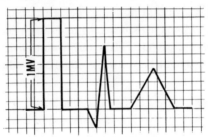

What Is an ECG
Lead Axis?

We assume in clinical electrocardiography that the QRS
and T deflections arise from a single point in the center of
the chest. This point, called E, is halfway between the
breastbone and the spine, and is thus in the exact center of
the thorax. From this point, electrical activity can proceed
in three different directions at once: left or right, down or
up, and front or back. It is quite evident that an electrical
impulse could be travelling to the left and also to the front
(anterior) at the same time. However, it could not be located to the left and to the right at the same time!

Let us consider the left-right relationship first. Lead I of
the electrocardiogram is a *left-right* lead. Any electrical
force, be it QRS or T, if directed to the *left,* results in an
upright (positive) deflection in the finished lead I record.
Any electrical activity directed to the *right* from the E
point results in a *downward* (negative) deflection in lead I
(Fig. 5).

The QRS and T shown in Figure 5 came from lead I (the
left-right lead). The deflections *below* the baseline (the Q
and the S) represent *rightward* electrical activity, whereas
the R wave and the T (positive deflections) represent

7

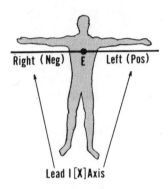

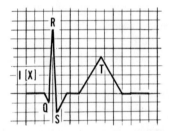

Fig. 5.—Lead I (*X*) axis. Note *QRS* and positive *T*. *R* and *T* are positive, or leftwards. *Q* and *S* are negative, or rightwards.

leftward activity. In this illustration, representing a QRS and T from a normal adult, *the major QRS deflection is directed to the left.* As shown, *the direction of T in a normal adult is also to the left.* Frequently, as in this case, small *initial* and *terminal* QRS forces (the Q and S) are directed to the *right.* (Some *normal* patients *lack* these initial and terminal *rightward* forces.)

In this text, the left-right lead axis will be called X. In the routine electrocardiographic tracings recorded daily in any hospital, or seen in textbooks, the lead which best reflects left and right (or X axis) forces is *lead I*.

Lead Y

Lead Y records only *downward* (inferior, footward) or *upward* (superior, headward) electrical activity. If an electrical force is directed *footwards* from the E point, the finished electrocardiogram in lead Y displays a positive deflection from the baseline. If electrical activity is directed *superiorly* from the E point, the finished electrocardiogram, in lead Y, will record a *negative* deflection. In the 12-lead electrocardiogram, *lead AVF* may be used as a Y lead axis.

Consider the normal adult lead AVF (Y) electrocardiographic record shown in Figure 6. Notice the small Q, tall R, small S, and upright T waves. In this case, since the lead recorded is lead AVF (or Y), the Q and S waves indicate *initial* and *terminal superior* QRS activity, while the *major* deflection (the R wave) indicates *footward* QRS activity. The T wave is clearly *footwards* or *inferior*.

Figure 6 illustrates a typical, normal lead AVF (or Y axis lead) and shows that the *major* QRS forces are normally *inferior* and that the T is also *inferior*. However, the initial and terminal QRS forces (Q and S) *may* be superior in relation to the E point. These initial and terminal (Q and S) *superior* QRS forces *may* well be absent in many normal subjects.

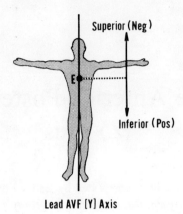

Lead AVF [Y] Axis

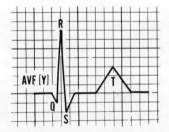

Fig. 6.–Lead *A VF* axis. Note *QRS* and positive *T. R* and *T* are positive, or inferior. *Q* and *S* are negative, or superior.

We have seen, so far, that the *normal human QRS* is directed mainly to the *left* and *inferior* and that the *T* is also directed *left* and *inferior*. The *initial* and *terminal* QRS forces, however, *may* be *rightward* and *superior*. Up to this point, we have characterized the QRS and T in *four* directions (*left-right* and *inferior-superior*), as defined by *two* lead axes (X, or lead I) and (Y, or lead AVF).

The Anterior-Posterior (Z) Axis

In this axis, best represented by lead V2 of the 12-lead electrocardiogram, forces directed *anteriorly* from the E point produce an *upright* deflection, while forces directed *posteriorly* produce a *negative* deflection. Figure 7 displays V2 recorded from a normal adult subject. Note the *RS* with *positive T*. In this normal record the *early* QRS forces are distinctly *anterior,* but the *major* QRS forces are posterior to the E point. The T wave is *anterior* in direction. This is the common, normal picture. It is *extremely unusual* for a normal patient to lack *any* early anterior QRS forces. It would also be unusual for the *anterior* QRS forces to be of *higher* magnitude than the *posterior* QRS forces.

Figure 8 presents a simultaneous display of XYZ leads in the normal subject. Note that the major QRS force is directed to the *left*-positive in lead I (X), *inferior*-positive in lead AVF (Y), and *posterior*-negative in lead V2 (Z). The early QRS forces are definitely *anterior*-upright in lead V2 (Z). Small, *rightwards*, initial and terminal QRS forces are present: Q and S wave in lead I (X). Initial and terminal *superior* QRS forces are also noted: Q and S wave in lead

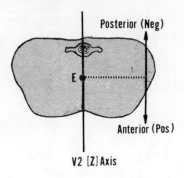

V2 [Z] Axis

Lead V₂ [Z] Axis

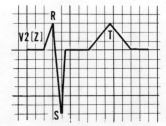

Fig. 7.–Note *RS* and positive *T*. *R* and *T* are anterior. *S* is posterior.

AVF (Y). The T deflections in this normal record are *left*-positive in lead I (X), *inferior*-positive in AVF (Y), and *anterior*-positive in V2 (Z).

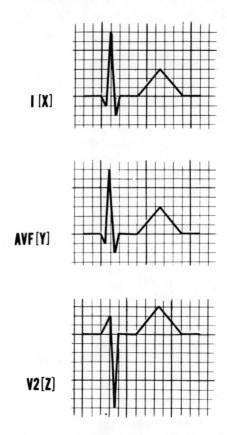

Fig. 8.—Normal *XYZ* electrocardiogram. The major QRS deflection is left-positive in *I (X)*, inferior-positive in *A VF (Y)*, and posterior-negative in *V2 (Z)*. Initial QRS forces are rightward-Q in *I (X)*, superior-Q in *A VF (Y)*, and anterior-R in *V2 (Z)*. T is left, inferior and anterior-positive in *I (X)*, *A VF (Y)*, and *V2 (Z)*.

The Ninety-Degree Rule

In electrocardiography, a QRS or T wave, beginning at the E point and directed to the *left,* for example, will produce the greatest voltage deflection in lead I (X) (Fig. 9). Such a wave (like A in Fig. 9) will be perpendicular to the lead AVF (Y) axis. Its effect upon the electrocardiogram recorded from lead axis AVF (Y) will be *very small.* The recorded electrocardiogram in lead AVF (Y) will show *small* or *zero* voltage.

In the same way (see Fig. 10), a QRS force directed *inferiorly* from the E point along the axis of lead AVF will produce a strong *upright* deflection in ECG lead AVF (Y). Because this electrical force is *perpendicular* to lead I (X), that lead will record a *small* or *zero* potential. When lead axes are *perpendicular* to each other—as leads I (X), AVF (Y), and V2 (Z) are, under ideal circumstances—they are said to be "orthogonal."

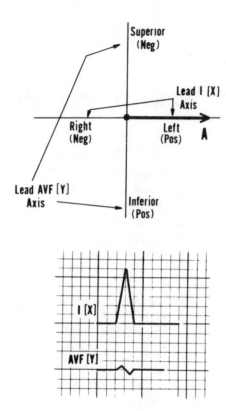

Fig. 9.—QRS wave *A* is directed left and therefore results in a positive deflection in *lead I (X)*. However, wave *A* is perpendicular (90°) to the *AVF (Y) axis,* and that lead records a small or zero deflection.

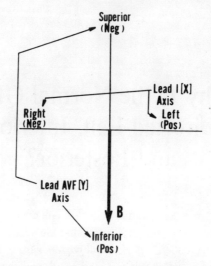

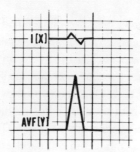

Fig. 10.—QRS wave *B* is directed inferiorly along the *AVF (Y) axis* and therefore produces a positive deflection in *AVF (Y)*. *B* is perpendicular to the *lead I (X) axis,* and that lead shows a small or zero deflection.

Why Is the Normal QRS Directed Left, Inferior and Posterior?

The normal X, Y, and Z leads that you are learning to recognize show, over and over again, that the normal QRS complex is directed *left, inferior,* and *posterior* from the E point. This is the anatomic and electrical position of the *left* ventricle of the heart.

Everyone knows that the normal blood pressure is about 120 mm of mercury. The left ventricle must pump against that pressure load. The right ventricle, on the other hand, pumps blood into a much lower pressure system, about 20 mm of mercury (Fig. 11). The ventricle working against the *higher* pressure load naturally becomes thicker. The thicker ventricle (the left one) produces *greater* QRS voltages. Therefore, in the normal subject, the electrical activity of the *right* ventricle is overshadowed by the thicker and stronger *left* ventricle. In this way the observed electrocardiogram in the normal subject is the electrocardiogram of the *left* ventricle, sometimes called a "levo" cardiogram.

The left and right ventricles contract at the same time and produce QRS complexes at the same time, because

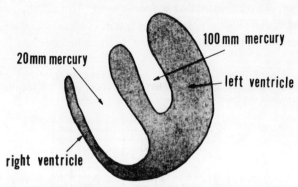

Fig. 11.—The *left ventricle* normally works against a much higher pressure load than the *right ventricle*. Consequently, the *left ventricle* is thicker and stronger than the *right* and dominates the normal electrocardiogram.

Fig. 12.—Normally, activation of *left* and *right ventricles* is simultaneous via the *bundle branches*. The QRS complex has a total duration of 0.10 seconds (100 milliseconds) or less.

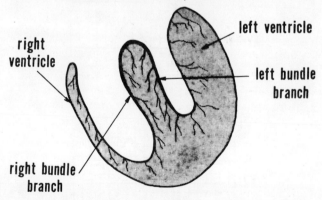

their electrical activation is *simultaneous*. This simultaneous activation (Figure 12) occurs by means of special conducting pathways in each ventricle called the "bundle branches."

Fig. 13.–The total QRS duration is two time boxes, or 0.08 seconds. Therefore, activation of left and right ventricles was simultaneous via the bundle branches.

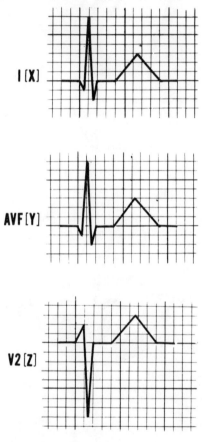

The special conducting pathway in the *right* ventricle is called the *"right bundle branch;"* the special conducting pathway in the *left* ventricle is called the *"left bundle branch."*

When electrical activation of *both* ventricles occurs *simultaneously* via this bundle branch system, the total duration of the QRS complex is 0.10 seconds (100 milliseconds) or less (Figure 13). Note that the total time duration from the beginning of the Q wave to the end of the S wave is two time boxes. Each time box represents 0.04 (1/25th) of a second. Therefore the total duration of this QRS complex is 0.08 seconds. This may also be expressed as 80 milliseconds. In this instance, since the duration of the QRS complex is 100 milliseconds or less, we may presume that the electrical activation of both ventricles occurred via the bundle-branch system, and that both bundle branches were functioning properly.

Left-Ventricular Hypertrophy

When the left ventricle enlarges beyond its normal size, the QRS voltage produced by the left ventricle *increases*. The magnitude of the *leftward,* and of the *posterior,* QRS voltages typically increases. The voltage in the AVF (Y) axis usually does *not* increase. This is because as the left ventricle enlarges, the anatomic and electrical axes become somewhat more *superior.* That is, the QRS forces are oriented more along the lead I (X) axis, and are therefore more perpendicular to the lead AVF (Y) axis than in the normal subject. Thus, although the *over-all* magnitude of the QRS complex may be *increased* in the leftward and posterior directions, it may actually *decrease* as recorded in the AVF (Y) axis. Remember the rule of the perpendicular!

In early left-ventricular hypertrophy, the T wave will remain in its normal position; that is, left-positive in lead I (X) and anterior-positive in lead V2 (Z). However, as left-ventricular hypertrophy advances, the T wave moves in a direction *opposite* the QRS complex, and ultimately will be found to the *right* of the E point: negative in lead I (X) and anterior-positive in lead V2 (Z). Figure 14 illustrates early left-ventricular hypertrophy. The amplitude of QRS in lead

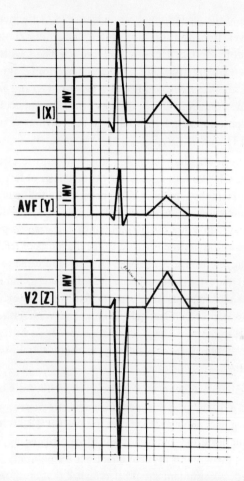

Fig. 14.—Early left-ventricular hypertrophy. The leftwards (*X axis*) and posterior *(Z axis)* QRS voltages are increased. The T direction remains normal (left, inferior, and anterior). Note half standardization (1 *mv* = 5 mm).

I (X) and the posterior voltage in lead V2 (Z) are increased. However, the T remains normal (*left* and *anterior*). In contrast, note the T deflections in Figure 15. Here, with a similar increase in leftward (X axis) and posterior (Z axis) QRS forces, the T is *rightward*-negative in lead I (X) and *anterior*-upright in lead V2 (Z). In this case, the left-ventricular hypertrophy is more advanced than in the previous example (Fig. 14).

Many studies have been done in an attempt to establish reliable QRS voltage criteria for the diagnosis of left-ventricular hypertrophy. In the XYZ approach, the following figures may prove useful. A *posterior* amplitude of 3 mv—that is, an S wave—in V2 (Z) of 30 mm indicates *increased* posterior voltage and therefore is a clue to the diagnosis of left-ventricular hypertrophy. A *leftward* (X axis) amplitude of 20 mm (2 mv) indicates increased leftward QRS forces, and is also a clue to the diagnosis of left-ventricular hypertrophy. If the QRS in lead I (X) is not quite 20 mm and V2 (Z) is not quite 30, but the sum of I (X), AVF (Y), and V2 (Z) voltages equals *50 mm,* left-ventricular hypertrophy should still be suspected.

Beginning students of electrocardiography, for whom this text is written, need *not* memorize absolute magnitudes. The beginner should realize that the *normal* QRS is located left and posterior, and that when left-ventricular hypertrophy occurs, the voltages in these directions are naturally increased. The student should also realize that in *severe* left-ventricular hypertrophy, the T wave is directed *opposite* the QRS, eventually coming to lie to the *right*-negative in lead I (X) and *anterior*-positive in V2 (Z).

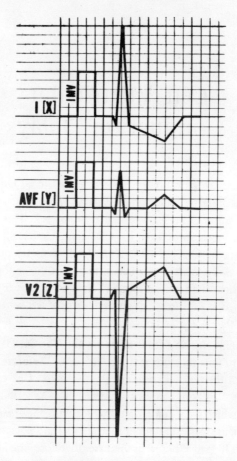

Fig. 15.—Advanced left-ventricular hypertrophy. In addition to increased left and posterior QRS voltage, the T is directed right and anterior, negative in *I (X)* and positive in *V2 (Z)*. Note half standardization (1 *mv* = 5 mm).

Left-Ventricular Conduction Delays

Sometimes activation of the left ventricle does *not* occur through the left-bundle-branch system. When this happens, the activation of the left ventricle is *prolonged*. This results in an *increased duration* of the QRS complex, usually to *three* time boxes, 0.12 seconds (120 milliseconds), or *even longer*. Since the *left* ventricle is the site of the abnormal conduction, the terminal forces of the QRS complex will be located in the directions characteristic of *left*-ventricular forces—that is, *left* and *posterior*.

Examine the XYZ leads in Figure 16. The QRS is prolonged to four time boxes (0.16 seconds). Therefore, activation of the ventricles was *not* simultaneous. One ventricle must be the site of abnormal conduction. The terminal QRS forces, which must come from the side with *abnormal* conduction, are leftward-upright in lead I (X) and posterior-negative in lead V2 (Z). In this case, therefore, the abnormal conduction must be located in the *left* ventricle.

There are three possible causes for abnormal left ventricular conduction: (1) left-bundle-branch block, (2) premature contractions arising in the right ventricle, and (3) pacemaker-induced complexes.

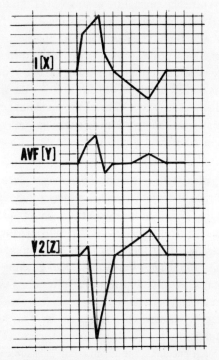

Fig. 16.—Left-ventricular conduction delay. The QRS duration, four time boxes (0.16 seconds), is abnormally long. The terminal QRS forces are left and posterior, indicating the left ventricle as the site of the conduction delay. The T wave in left-ventricular conduction delay is right and anterior-negative T in *I (X)* and positive T in *V2 (Z)*.

1. A block in the *left*-bundle-branch system may occur, preventing transmission of the electrical impulse along this specialized conducting pathway. This is called "left-bundle-branch block."

2. A ventricular premature beat, arising from the *opposite* (right) ventricle will *also* result in abnormal *left*-ventricular conduction. The reason is this: the electrical impulse begins someplace in the *right* ventricle, then spreads across the muscular septum separating the two ventricles, and enters the left ventricle *without* utilizing the specialized *left*-bundle-branch system. Therefore, premature contractions arising from the *right* ventricle exhibit "left-ventricular conduction delay" and closely resemble the QRS complexes of *left*-bundle-branch block.

3. A patient with an *electrical pacemaker* placed in the *right* ventricle undergoes a sequence of events closely resembling that described for *right*-ventricular premature contractions. The electrical stimulus *first* activates the *right* ventricle. Then, after spreading through the muscular septum, it activates the *left* ventricle *without* entering the left-bundle-branch system. In this way, the resulting QRS complex is prolonged, because the *left* ventricle is abnormally activated. The terminal QRS forces are again oriented to the *left*-upright in lead I (X) and *posterior*-negative in lead V2 (Z). Such pacemaker-induced complexes are easy to identify because they are preceded by typical pacemaker "spikes."

Figures 17, 18, and 19 present electrocardiograms illustrating the three causes of abnormal left-ventricular conduction described above. In Figure 17, characteristic pacemaker spikes are followed by prolonged QRS complexes. The terminal QRS forces are leftward-upright in lead I (X) and *posterior*-negative in lead V2 (Z). Thus, in Figure 17 the correct diagnosis is *left-ventricular conduction delay* on the basis of *pacemaker stimuli* applied to the *right ventricle*.

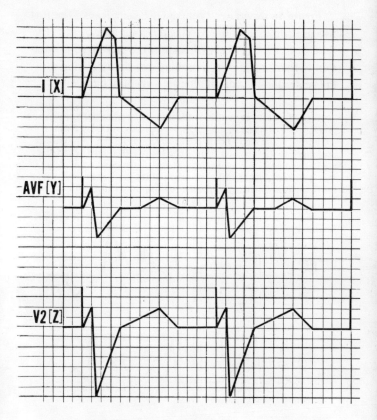

Fig. 17.—Right-ventricular pacing (causing left-ventricular conduction delay). QRS duration of four time boxes (0.16 seconds) is abnormally prolonged. Terminal QRS forces are left and posterior, indicating left-ventricular abnormal conduction. Note the pacemaker spikes and the right, anterior T.

Figure 18 shows *two* types of QRS complexes. The first two beats in each of the X, Y, and Z leads are normal. The third beat, which is early (premature), is *prolonged* in duration to *four* time boxes, indicating that the activation of the ventricles was *not* simultaneous via both bundle

Fig. 18.—Left-ventricular conduction delay from right-ventricular premature beat. The first two QRS complexes and their T waves are normal. The next QRS is premature (early). This third QRS is prolonged to 0.16 seconds (four time boxes). Terminal QRS forces are left and posterior, indicating left-ventricular conduction delay in that beat and a right-ventricular origin of the premature beat. Note the T, right-negative in *I (X)* and anterior-positive in *V2 (Z)*.

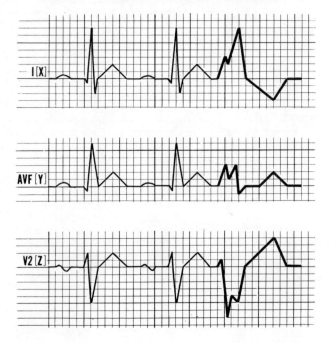

branches *in that beat*. The QRS is *prolonged* with the terminal forces again *left* and *posterior*. This indicates left-ventricular conduction delay, in this case on the basis of a premature contraction arising *spontaneously* in the right ventricle.

Figure 19 presents an electrocardiogram in which all the QRS complexes are prolonged, with the terminal forces again left and posterior. No beats are premature, and no pacing artifacts are seen. This is an example of *left-bundle-branch block*.

Now observe the T deflections in Figures 17, 18, and 19. Note that in *all three* types of left-ventricular conduction delay, the T wave is rightwards-negative in lead I (X) and anterior-upright in lead V2 (Z).

Fig. 19.—Left-bundle-branch block. All QRS complexes are prolonged beyond 0.12 seconds. The terminal QRS forces are left and posterior, indicating the conduction defect to be left ventricular. No beats are premature, and there are no pacing spikes. The cause of the left-ventricular conduction delay is left-bundle-branch block. As in other causes of left-ventricular conduction delay, T is right and anterior.

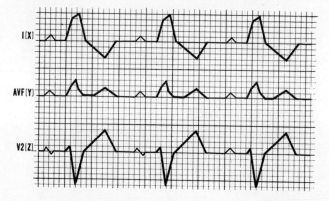

The preceding sections have been devoted to examples of *left-ventricular domination* of the electrocardiogram as a result of *left-ventricular hypertrophy* or *left-ventricular conduction delay*. Separation of the two is generally easy. In left-ventricular hypertrophy, QRS voltage is *increased* leftwards and posterior, but the QRS *duration* is within normal limits, although often at the upper limit. In the left-ventricular conduction delays, the QRS is *prolonged*, usually beyond 0.12 seconds, and the QRS voltage is often normal. Once the diagnosis of left-ventricular conduction delay has been established, one may recognize pacing spikes (which indicate right-ventricular pacing), or prematurity of the beats (which indicates a right-ventricular origin of the premature contraction), or neither of these, in which case left-bundle-branch block is usually the diagnosis.

In all of these electrocardiograms, in which the left ventricle dominates by virtue of hypertrophy or conduction delay, the T wave is located to the *right* and *anterior* of the E point.

The Right Ventricle

As pointed out in previous sections, the normal human adult electrocardiogram is dominated by *left*-ventricular forces because the work load of the *left* ventricle is normally five times that of the *right* ventricle. Under certain circumstances, the work load of the *right* ventricle may increase, with subsequent thickening (or hypertrophy) of the right-ventricular wall. At the same time, the *left ventricle* may remain unchanged or even decrease in its work load and size.

A clue to the electrical orientation of the right ventricle may be seen in the electrocardiogram of a newborn child (Figure 20). Here, the QRS in lead I (X) displays *prominent rightward* (negative) deflections, and the QRS in lead V2 (Z) is *predominantly anterior* (upright). Because the circulation of the unborn child is maintained almost exclusively by the *right* ventricle, *this* ventricle bears most of the work load and it therefore exceeds the left ventricle in size. Not surprisingly, then, in the *adult* human who develops right-ventricular hypertrophy, QRS forces are added which are located to the *right* and *anterior* to the E point.

Additional details are necessary at this point. When *rightward* forces are added to the QRS forces in right-ventricular hypertrophy, they are characteristically added

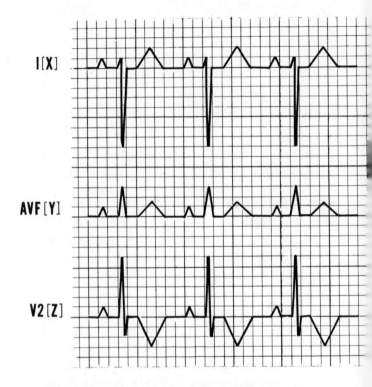

Fig. 20.—Physiologic right-ventricular hypertrophy in a newborn infant. Note prominent late rightwards QRS forces, deep S in lead *I (X)*; note also prominent early anterior QRS forces, tall R in *V2 (Z)*. T is left and posterior: positive in *I (X)* and negative in *V2 (Z)*.

in the *middle* and *terminal* portions of the QRS complex. Thus, the magnitude of the leftward QRS deflection in lead I (X) may be *reduced* while the magnitude of the terminal *rightward* QRS forces is greatly increased. On the other hand, when QRS forces are added *anteriorly* in right-ventricular hypertrophy, this addition is characteristically *early* rather than late. Thus, in these cases, the height of the R wave will increase in lead V2 (Z). Since no significant addition occurs in the *superior* or *inferior* QRS forces, lead AVF (Y) characteristically shows no QRS change in right-ventricular hypertrophy.

Figure 21 illustrates right-ventricular hypertrophy manifesting itself as a *late* addition of rightward forces. Note

Fig. 21.—Right-ventricular hypertrophy ("late rightward type"). The addition of middle and late rightwards QRS forces has reduced the magnitude of leftwards QRS forces; there is a small R in *I (X)* and a prominent S wave in *I (X)*. QRS in *AVF (Y)* and *V2 (Z)* remains normal. T is left and posterior-positive in *I (X)* and negative in *V2 (Z)*.

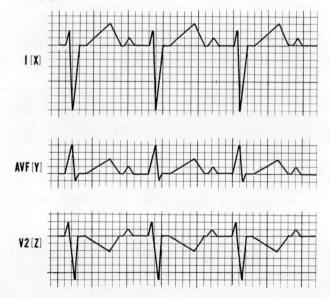

the prominent late rightward (S) wave in lead I (X), and the normal-appearing QRS complexes in lead AVF (Y) and lead V2 (Z). Note the direction of the T wave. It is leftward-upright in lead I (X). This is quite characteristic of the T direction in right-ventricular hypertrophy. Very often, the T is also *posterior* (especially in more severe right-ventricular hypertrophy), producing a negative T deflection in lead V2 (Z). In other cases, however, the T may be left but *anterior*-upright in lead V2 (Z).

Figure 22 illustrates the "anterior" type of right-ventricular hypertrophy. The QRS complexes in lead I (X) and lead AVF (Y) are normal. However, note the *prominent anterior* QRS forces in lead V2 (Z). Note also the decrease in the posterior QRS forces (the smaller S wave) in lead V2 (Z). The T wave, however, is again leftward-upright in lead I (X).

One of the curious things about right-ventricular hypertrophy is that two successive patients with identical conditions leading to right-ventricular hypertrophy (for example, obstruction of the pulmonary valve, or mitral valve stenosis) may present quite different electrocardiographic profiles. One patient may have the *rightward* type of right-ventricular hypertrophy with the addition of late rightward forces, while the second patient shows the *anterior* type of right-ventricular hypertrophy, with only the *early* addition of *anterior* forces. In both instances, however, the *T* will be directed to the *left*.

In the most severe cases, *both* abnormalities illustrated in Figures 21 and 22 occur simultaneously. That is, *rightward* forces will be added in the *middle* and *terminal* portions of the QRS, and *anterior* forces will be added *especially early*

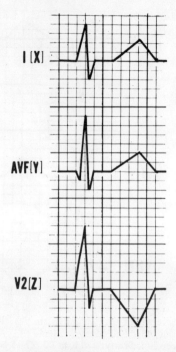

Fig. 22.—Right-ventricular hypertrophy ("early anterior type"). Addition of early anterior QRS forces is recorded in *V2 (Z)* as a tall R wave. The posterior QRS forces, S wave in *V2 (Z)*, are reduced. QRS in *I (X)* and *AVF (Y)* is not affected. T is left-positive in *I (X)* and posterior-negative in *V2 (Z)*.

to the QRS complexes. When this occurs, the diagnosis of right-ventricular hypertrophy is easy. Figure 23 is an example of right-ventricular hypertrophy displaying both *late rightward* and *early anterior* QRS forces, with a characteristic *left* and *posterior* T wave.

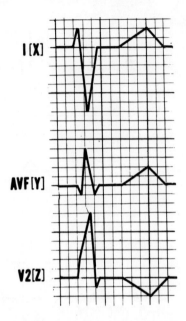

Fig. 23.—Severe right-ventricular hypertrophy. Rightwards QRS forces have been added late: deep S in lead *I (X)*. Anterior QRS forces have been added early: tall R in *V2 (Z)*. T is left-positive in *I (X)* and posterior-negative in *V2 (Z)*.

You may have noticed that the QRS duration in these examples of right ventricular hypertrophy is *not* prolonged. That is, the duration of the QRS complexes is two and one-half time boxes or less (0.10 seconds or less). This is because conduction through the right- and left-bundle-branch systems is simultaneous.

Right-Ventricular Conduction Delays

When the activation of the *right* ventricle is *abnormal* (*not* through the *right* bundle branch), the QRS complex is prolonged to 0.12 seconds (three time boxes) or more. Since the *right* ventricle is the site of delay, the terminal QRS forces are oriented in the typical directions for *right*-ventricular QRS forces, that is, to the *right* and *anterior* of the E point. Thus, in *right*-ventricular conduction delay, the terminal QRS forces will be negative in lead I (X) (an S wave) and usually positive (an R') in lead V2 (Z). This terminal QRS force may be *inferior* or *superior* (positive or negative) in lead AVF (Y), which therefore is *not* a useful guide to the diagnosis of *right*-ventricular conduction delay.

In *right*-ventricular conduction delays, the T is located in the same direction characteristic for *right*-ventricular hypertrophy. That is, the T will be to the *left* of the E point: upright in lead I (X) and either posterior-negative in lead V2 (Z) or anterior-upright in lead V2 (Z).

Right ventricular conduction delays are of three types: (1) right-bundle-branch block, (2) electrical pacing of the left ventricle, and (3) premature left-ventricular contraction.

1. In *right-bundle-branch block,* the cardiac rhythm is undisturbed by premature beats, but the QRS complex is prolonged (Figure 24). Note that the terminal QRS forces are oriented to the *right*-negative in lead I (X) and *anterior*-positive in lead V2 (Z). The T is *leftwards*-upright in lead I (X) and *posterior*-negative in lead V2 (Z). The QRS complex is prolonged to 140 milliseconds (0.14 seconds, or three and one-half time boxes). The diagnosis here is *right-ventricular conduction delay* on the basis of *right-bundle-branch block.*

2. Another cause of *right*-ventricular conduction delay is electrical pacing of the *left* ventricle. If the pacing

Fig. 24.–Right-bundle-branch block. QRS is prolonged to three and one-half time boxes, or 0.14 seconds. Terminal QRS forces are right-S in lead *I (X)* and anterior-R' in *V2 (Z)*. This localizes the delay to the right ventricle. The QRS complexes are not premature. No pacing spikes are noted. T is left-positive in *I (X)* and posterior-negative in *V2 (Z)*.

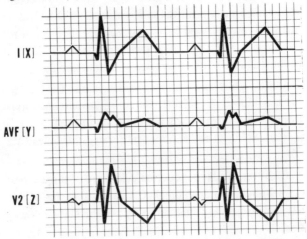

stimulus is applied to the *left* ventricle, *that* ventricle writes its QRS complex *first*. The electrical impulse then spreads across the septum and through the right ventricle, but *not* through the right-bundle-branch system. This *prolongs* the QRS complex with *right*-ventricular conduction delay. The terminal QRS forces are again oriented to the *right* and *anterior,* and the T wave is again oriented to the *left* and usually *posterior*. Such cases can be easily identified, because the prolonged QRS complexes, with their terminal forces oriented to the *right* and *anterior,* are preceded by typical pacing artifacts. In Figure 25, the QRS complexes are prolonged to 0.16 seconds. This indicates a ventricular conduction delay. The terminal forces are oriented to the *right*-negative in lead I (X) and *anterior*-positive in lead V2 (Z). The T deflection is to the *left*-upright in lead I (X). This all indicates a *right*-ventricular conduction delay. Since each QRS complex is preceded by a *pacing spike,* the diagnosis of a pacemaker mechanism is evident. Because the conduction delay is clearly in the *right* ventricle, the pacemaker stimuli are applied to the *left* ventricle.

3. Right-ventricular conduction delay may also be caused by a premature ventricular contraction arising from the *left* ventricle. In this instance (Figure 26), instead of a *pacing spike* applied to the left ventricle, *a spontaneous* focus stimulates the left ventricle. *In that beat,* the *left* ventricle therefore writes its QRS complex first, and the activation wave again spreads across the septum to the right ventricle, *not utilizing* the *right*-bundle-branch pathway. QRS prolongation results, with the terminal QRS forces again oriented *right* and *anterior*. The T wave is again oriented to the *left*-positive in lead I (X), and usually *posterior*-negative in lead

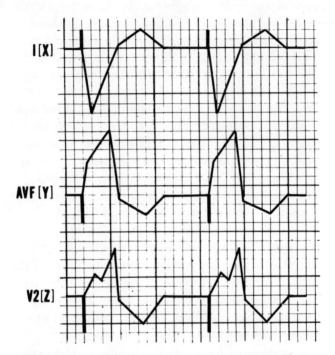

Fig. 25.–Left-ventricular pacing, producing right-ventricular conduction delay. QRS is prolonged to four time boxes (0.16 seconds).
Terminal QRS forces are right-S wave in *I (X)* and anterior-R′ in *V2
(Z)*, indicating right-ventricular delay. Each QRS is preceded by a
pacemaker artifact. T is left-positive in *I (X)* and posterior-negative
in *V2 (Z)*.

V2 (Z). In Figure 26, the *third* beat is characteristically
prolonged to 140 milliseconds with terminal forces to the
right, indicating a right-ventricular conduction delay. However, the beat is clearly earlier than expected from the heart
rhythm, indicating that it is a premature contraction. The

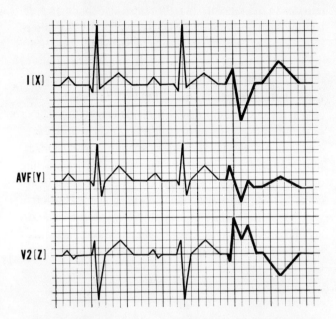

Fig. 26.–Right-ventricular conduction delay in a premature beat of left-ventricular origin. After two normal beats, a premature QRS of prolonged duration (0.16 seconds) occurs. Terminal QRS forces in that beat are right-S in *I (X)* and anterior-R′ in *V2 (Z)*, indicating right-ventricular delay. T is left-positive in *I (X)* and posterior-negative in *V2 (Z)*.

diagnosis in this case is a premature ventricular contraction arising from the *left* ventricle and presenting with *right-*ventricular conduction delay.

In summary, when the *right* ventricle dominates the electrocardiogram, either through *right-ventricular hypertrophy or right-ventricular conduction delay,* the QRS forces become increasingly evident to the *right* of the E point and *anterior* to the E point. In *right*-ventricular conduction delay, the total duration of the QRS complex is 120 milliseconds or more. In right-ventricular hypertrophy, the QRS duration is normal (100 milliseconds, or less). In all of these conditions, the T is directed to the *left,* usually *posterior,* but sometimes *anterior.* Lead AVF (Y) is not valuable in the diagnosis of right-ventricular conduction delay or right-ventricular hypertrophy. When right-ventricular conduction delay is diagnosed, an attempt should be made to determine the *nature* of the right-ventricular conduction delay. A *pacing spike* preceding the QRS complexes indicates that the pacemaker stimulus was applied to the left ventricle. A *premature* beat exhibiting *right*-ventricular delay indicates a *left*-ventricular origin of the beat. Absence of both of these indicates right-bundle-branch block.

Myocardial Infarction:
"Infarction Means Subtraction"

In the sections on right- and left-ventricular hypertrophy, we have seen how *addition* of QRS forces to the *left* and *posterior* (in the case of left-ventricular hypertrophy) or *right* and *anterior* (in the case of right-ventricular hypertrophy) can change the QRS complexes. When areas of the *left* ventricle are damaged by heart attacks (or myocardial infarctions), QRS forces are *subtracted* from the damaged areas. This subtraction may occur *at any time* during the QRS cycle, depending on the location of the damaged muscle. In the case of damage to the *anterior wall* of the left ventricle, or to the *inferior wall* of the left ventricle, such subtraction occurs *early* in the QRS complex, usually in the first 0.04 seconds (40 milliseconds).

Anterior Infarction

Let us first consider the effects of *anterior* infarction on the QRS complex. Since the normal early QRS forces are *anterior* in position, producing an R wave in lead V2 (Z), this is the lead which will show the greatest change in *anterior* infarction. Characteristically, in an anterior infarction, these normal anterior QRS forces are "subtracted" or lost. They are greatly reduced or simply *disappear*. Therefore the R (anterior) forces in lead V2 (Z) may be no longer seen, and lead V2 will present itself as a "Q-S" complex (entirely negative, or *posterior*).

If the damaged muscle, before infarction, had produced *only* anterior QRS forces, no change at all would occur in the left-right or inferior-superior QRS forces recorded in lead I (X) or lead AVF (Y). The QRS complexes in lead I (X) and AVF (Y), therefore, would be entirely normal. Figure 27 shows normal-appearing QRS complexes in lead I (X) and in lead AVF (Y). But note the absence of R waves in lead V2 (Z). This *loss* of the normally early anterior QRS forces is consistent with the "subtraction" effect of anterior myocardial infarction.

Areas of infarction may affect more than the QRS complex of the electrocardiogram. Infarcts may include *ischemic* zones. An ischemic zone *repolarizes* (recharges) relatively

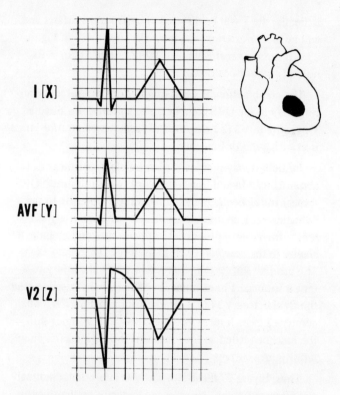

Fig. 27.—Anterior infarction. Anterior muscle necrosis resulted in loss of normal anterior QRS forces: absent R in *V2 (Z)*. Anterior ischemia means slow repolarization in that area, with T directed away: posterior or negative T in *V2 (Z)*. Anterior injury causes an anterior baseline shift after the QRS: ST elevated in *V2 (Z)*. Leads *I (X)* and *AVF (Y)* are not affected.

later than uninvolved, normal tissue. Consequently, the T will be directed *away* from such ischemic zones. In the case of *anterior* infarction, for example, with areas of *anterior*

ischemia, the T will be directed *away* from the infarct and
will be more *posterior* than normal. Thus the T in Figure
27 is posterior-*negative* in lead V2 (Z), rather than in its
normal *anterior* position.

The combination of a loss of *anterior* QRS forces occurring *early* in the QRS complex, plus a *posteriorly* directed
T-negative in V2 (Z) suggests the diagnosis of *anterior* infarction with *anterior* ischemia.

Infarction may present yet a third electrocardiographic
abnormality. In addition to *necrosis* (which subtracts QRS
forces) and *ischemia* (which directs the T opposite to the
ischemic area), an infarcted area may produce *injury currents.* Injury currents appear in the electrocardiogram as a
change in the *baseline* which *follows* the QRS complex.
The baseline shift is *in the direction* where the injury current is located. For example, in Figure 27 the baseline *after*
the QRS in lead V2 (Z) is clearly displaced *anteriorly* when
compared to its level *before* the QRS. This *anterior* shift of
the baseline (called an "S-T segment shift") indicates an *anterior* injury current.

Thus, Figure 27 illustrates *all three* infarction abnormalities discussed so far. *Necrosis* led to a subtraction of early
anterior QRS forces, resulting in the loss of the initial R
wave in lead V2 (Z). *Ischemia* is also present, which directs
the T in an abnormally *posterior* direction, resulting in a
negative T in lead V2 (Z). Lastly, an *injury current* is present, which shifts the baseline *after* the QRS complex in an
anterior direction. Because all of these changes occurred
along *one axis* of the electrocardiogram (the Z axis) the
changes are most clearly seen in *lead V2* which may be used
as a Z axis lead. Lead I (X) and lead AVF (Y) of the electrocardiogram show little or no change.

Inferior Infarction

Infarction may occur in muscle whose activity is recorded along the AVF (Y) axis, as well. When *inferior* infarction occurs, the characteristic changes of necrosis (QRS subtraction), ischemia (T wave redirection), and injury current (S-T baseline shift) are most characteristically seen in the AVF (Y) axis of the electrocardiogram. The Y axis is *not* very useful in the diagnosis of left-ventricular hypertrophy, left-ventricular conduction defects, right-ventricular hypertrophy, or right-ventricular conduction defects. However, the AVF (Y) axis is *extremely* valuable in the diagnosis of inferior infarction.

Figure 28 shows the abnormalities in lead AVF (Y). Although small initial superior forces in lead AVF (Y) may be normal (Q wave), in this instance the Q wave is of *abnormally prolonged* duration (about 40 milliseconds, or one full time box) and the amplitude of the Q wave is greater than 25% of the following R wave. These are useful criteria which help separate a normal Q wave in lead AVF (Y) from an *abnormal* one which indicates the *subtraction* effect of an inferior infarction. The abnormal superior initial deflection in lead AVF (Y) results from necrosis of muscle located in the AVF (Y) axis and contributing *early* to the QRS complex. Thus, the loss (subtraction) of this muscle results in an *upward* (superior) deflection in the finished electrocardiogram in lead AVF (Y).

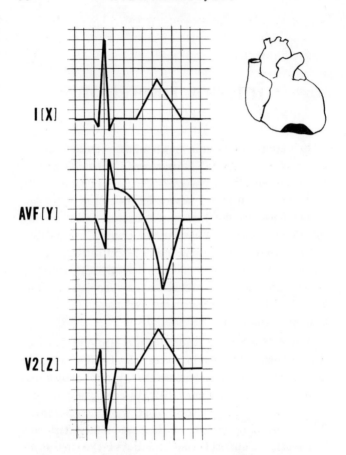

Fig. 28.–Inferior infarction. Inferior muscle necrosis subtracts early QRS forces in the *AVF (Y)* axis, resulting in increased early superior QRS forces: Q in lead *AVF (Y)*. Inferior ischemia means slow repolarization in that area with T directed away or superior-negative T in lead *AVF (Y)*. Inferior injury currents shift the *AVF (Y)* baseline inferiorly after the QRS: ST elevated in lead *AVF (Y)*. Leads *I (X)* and *V2 (Z)* are not affected.

This area of necrosis may be surrounded by an area of ischemia. The repolarization (recharging) of this ischemic tissue is *slower* than the repolarization in other areas. Therefore, the T wave is directed *away* from the ischemic tissue. A strongly negative (superior) T in lead AVF (Y) results.

The area of infarction may also produce *injury currents.* This results in a new baseline after the QRS complex. In Figure 28, illustrating inferior infarction, this change of baseline is clearly directed *inferiorly* and upwards in lead AVF (Y). Thus the QRS, T, and S-T abnormalities all *localize* the area of damage to the *inferior* area of the heart. Note, though, that the lead I (X) axis is normal. The Z axis (V2) may also be completely normal in inferior infarction. However, since ischemia of the *posterior* (dorsal) wall is often associated with inferior infarction, commonly the T wave will be *more* anterior than normal, resulting in a *more positive* T in lead V2 (Z) than in the normal case.

We emphasize again that inferior infarction is one of the few conditions in which the AVF (Y) axis plays an important diagnostic role.

So far, we have considered *anterior* infarction and *inferior* infarction. In each of these, the subtraction effect of the muscle necrosis occurred *early* in the QRS cycle. In the case of *anterior* infarction, this subtraction resulted in a loss of normal *anterior* forces, and in the case of inferior infarction in a loss of early *inferior* forces.

Lateral Infarction

Lateral infarction is best seen in the X axis of the electro-cardiogram. QRS subtraction from lateral wall necrosis may take place *early* in the QRS complex, in the *middle* of the QRS complex, or sometimes even *late* in the QRS complex (or in some combination of these). When the subtraction of leftward (X axis) forces occurs early, the normal initial rightward QRS force (Q in lead X or I) is *prolonged* and *deepened.* When the subtraction occurs in the *middle* of the QRS complex, the *height* of the *R wave* (leftward deflection) in lead I (X) is reduced. When the QRS subtraction from the lateral wall occurs *late,* the normal S wave (rightward force) in lead I (X) *increases,* producing a *deeper S wave* in that lead.

Figures 29, 30, and 31 show three examples of lateral in-farction. In Figure 29, the QRS subtraction is largely *early,* resulting in a deep Q wave in lead I (X). In Figure 30, the subtraction is both early and middle. Note the marked *re-duction* in the *R wave* (smaller leftward forces). And in Figure 31, note the *late subtraction*, producing a deep S wave in lead I (X). In each of these examples, the T wave in lead X is strongly rightward (negative). This reflects *late* repolarization of the lateral wall (*lateral ischemia*). In all

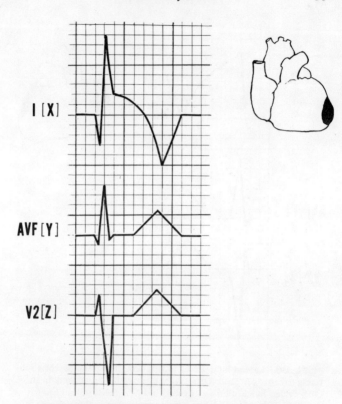

Fig. 29.–Lateral infarction. In this case, the QRS subtraction due to lateral necrosis is early, causing increased magnitude of early rightward QRS forces: Q in *I (X)*. Lateral ischemia (slow lateral wall repolarization) directs the T right (away from the ischemic zone). Note negative T in *I (X)*. Lateral injury currents shift the baseline after the QRS to the left: ST shifted left, or positively, in *I (X)*. Leads *AVF (Y)* and *V2 (Z)* are not affected.

three cases, the baseline *after* the QRS complex is *elevated* indicating lateral *injury currents* as well.

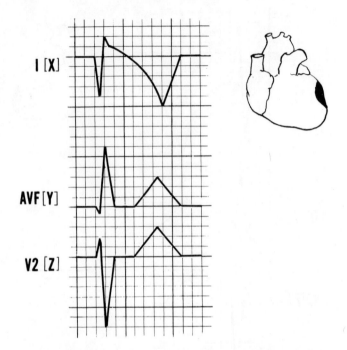

Fig. 30.—Lateral infarction. In this case, the lateral necrosis subtracts leftwards *(X)* axis QRS forces both early and midway in the QRS cycle. In addition to a deep Q in *I (X)*, the R in lead *I (X)* is reduced. Ischemic and injury effects are similar to those shown in Figure 29.

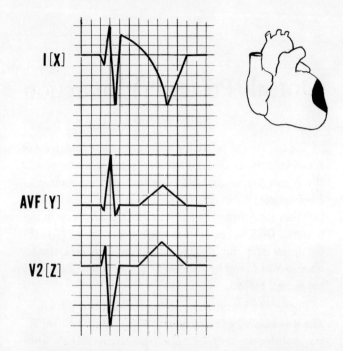

Fig. 31.–Lateral infarction. Lateral necrosis in this case results in late leftwards subtraction from QRS, producing prominent late rightward QRS forces: deep S in lead *I (X)*. Ischemic (T wave) and injury (ST shift) effects are the same as those in Figure 29.

Dorsal (Posterior) Infarction

The last area of infarction to be discussed is *posterior* or *dorsal* infarction. QRS subtraction from the posterior wall also occurs *later* in the QRS cycle than does subtraction from the *anterior* or *inferior* wall. The result is an increase in the *anterior forces:* taller R in V2 (Z), a *decrease* in the posterior QRS forces, with a smaller S wave in V2 (Z). If the dorsal infarction also includes an *ischemic* area, the T wave in V2 (Z) will be more *anterior* (more upright) than in the normal subject.

Figure 32 illustrates normal-appearing X and Y leads. The R in lead V2 (Z) is markedly *increased* (prominent R wave) with a markedly *anterior* T-positive in V2 (Z). The S-T shift after the QRS in V2 (Z) is negative, indicating a *posterior* injury current. This ECG picture is *suggestive* of dorsal infarction.

The diagnosis of dorsal infarction is one of the most *difficult* and *unreliable* ECG diagnoses. When prominent *anterior* QRS forces, together with a prominently anterior T, are the *only* ECG abnormalities seen, the cardiologist may *suspect* true dorsal infarction, uncomplicated by inferior, or lateral infarction. However, this suspicion has been confirmed by anatomic or x-ray studies of coronary arteries in only about 60% of such cases. In other words, this

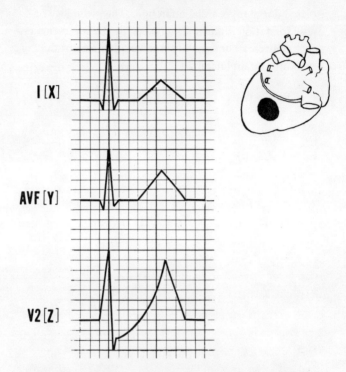

Fig. 32.—Dorsal (posterior) infarction. Posterior necrosis subtracts QRS forces from the posterior wall, increasing the amplitude of the normal anterior QRS forces: tall R in *V2 (Z)*. Posterior ischemia shifts the T more anterior than normal: T tall in *V2 (Z)*. Posterior injury currents shift the baseline (after the QRS) in a posterior direction: ST depressed or negative in lead *V2 (Z)*. Leads *I (X)* and *AVF (Y)* are not affected. Note: the diagnosis of posterior infarction is greatly strengthened if necrosis, ischemia, or injury can be demonstrated in lateral or inferior areas.

diagnosis may be *wrong* as often as 40% of the time. Therefore, great caution must be used in the diagnosis of true, isolated dorsal myocardial infarction. The possibility of dorsal infarction is much higher when the ECG presents evidence of necrosis or ischemia in some other area of the heart (inferior, or lateral).

Combined Myocardial Infarction

In most clinical cases of myocardial infarction, the areas of necrosis, injury, and ischemia affect *more* than one lead axis of the electrocardiogram. Anterior and lateral infarctions commonly coexist. Dorsal and lateral infarctions are another common combination. Inferior and lateral, inferior dorsal, or inferior and anterior infarctions also occur together with some frequency.

Figure 33 shows QRS (subtraction) abnormalities of infarction recorded in lead AVF (Y), while T changes of ischemia are noted in the X axis; the negative T in lead I (X) indicates lateral ischemia. Many combinations of necrosis, ischemia, or injury, each occurring in one, two, or three axes, are possible. Very often, the QRS changes of an infarction will persist for years. Then the patient may experience a fresh ischemic episode and develop T abnormalities in a *different* axis at a later date.

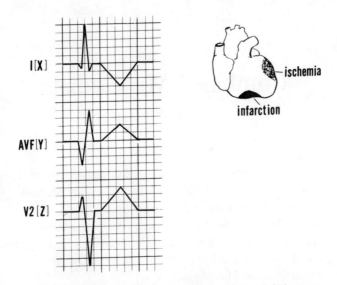

Fig. 33.—Inferior infarction with lateral ischemia. Inferior necrosis results in abnormal early superior QRS forces: deep Q in *AVF (Y)*. Lateral ischemia causes slow lateral repolarization, and the normally leftwards T is direct right: T negative in *I (X)*. Lead *V2 (Z)* is not affected.

False-Positive Infarction Diagnosis

Probably the most common error made in electrocardiographic diagnosis is the *overdiagnosis* of *anterior* infarction in patients with *left*-ventricular hypertrophy. As we have pointed out previously in this handbook, in *left*-ventricular hypertrophy QRS forces are added to the *left* and *posterior*. This increases the QRS voltage of R in lead I (X) axis and of S in lead V2 (Z) axis. If the *posterior* addition of QRS forces occurs *very early*, the anterior QRS forces, which were normally present, may *completely disappear*. This results in the *absence* of an R wave in lead V2 (Z), *simulating* an anterior infarction.

In patients studied by coronary arteriography (x-rays of the coronary arteries) who have left-ventricular hypertrophy with *absent anterior* QRS forces, the coronary arteries are found to be *completely normal* in 50% of the cases. Thus, caution is required in the diagnosis of anterior infarction when the patient has coexisting *left*-ventricular hypertrophy.

Pitfalls in Diagnosis When Right-Bundle-Branch Block Is Present

As pointed out previously, *right*-bundle-branch block prolongs the QRS complex because of *right*-ventricular conduction delay. The QRS complex is 120 milliseconds (three time boxes) or more in duration, with the terminal forces oriented to the *right* and *anterior.* When this *rightward* and *anterior* position occurs throughout the QRS complex, one is tempted to suspect the presence of *right-ventricular hypertrophy* also. This suspicion is frequently *unjustified.* It is true that patients with right-ventricular hypertrophy *may* manifest right-bundle-branch block. However, when right-bundle-branch block is present in patients *without* right-ventricular hypertrophy, the entire QRS complex may be *markedly* right and anterior. Thus, the ECG reader must be aware of the danger of *overdiagnosis* if he attempts to diagnose *right-ventricular hypertrophy* in the *presence* of *right-bundle-branch block.*

Another pitfall, when right-bundle-branch block is present, is the diagnosis of *true dorsal myocardial infarction.* We have already pointed out that the diagnosis of true dorsal myocardial infarction is dangerous enough in the *absence* of right-bundle-branch block. In the presence of *right-bundle-branch block,* this diagnosis is even *more* difficult. The reason is that right-bundle-branch block, *by itself,* can displace the QRS complexes in an *anterior direction* (in the same direction that *dorsal infarction* displaces the QRS complex).

The direction of the T wave is a *better* guide to dorsal wall damage than is the QRS complex, when right-bundle-branch block is present. A markedly anterior T, strongly upright in V2 (Z) and low in lead I (X), because it is almost perpendicular to lead I (X), in the presence of *right*-bundle-branch block, suggests dorsal-lateral ischemia. However, the diagnosis of muscle *necrosis* (infarction) in the dorsal wall, in the *presence* of right-bundle-branch block, is extremely difficult and frequently incorrect.

The ECG Secret

If there is a secret in understanding the electrocardiogram, it is simply this: one must learn to *translate* positive or negative deflections in leads I (X), AVF (Y), and V2 (Z) into *directions.* One should not refer to a "Q wave in lead X." One should think and say "an initial rightward force." One should not refer to a "high voltage S wave in lead V2," but should think and say "increased posterior voltage."

By constant translation of *deflections* into *directions,* the student of electrocardiography will learn to think in *six directions* along the three axes *(X, Y, and Z).* Unfortunately, leads I, AVF, and V2 are not *truly* X, Y, and Z leads. The AVF lead is *very* often a true Y axis lead, but leads I and V2 are *very* often *not* true X and Z axis leads.

Since the X and Z axes are the most valuable in ECG diagnosis, much research has been done to develop "electrode networks" which will produce perfect X, Y, and Z axis leads. Because most medical students, nurses, and technicians work and study in hospitals *not* using such networks, however, the best way for most beginners to start is by using leads I, AVF, and V2, described in this manual as X, Y, and Z leads.

This little book will close as it began. It is impossible to learn ECG interpretation from any instruction manual. The only way to learn is to find an expert, sit at his side for a period of three to six months, and absorb his knowledge on a day-to-day basis.

Suggested Readings

The interested student may wish to continue his study of ECG beyond the fundamentals described in this handbook. The following brief list of books will introduce him to basic and well-written texts on electrocardiography.

Chou, T. C., and Helm, R. A.: *Clinical Vectorcardiography* (New York and London: Grune & Stratton, Inc., 1967).

Dubin, D.: *Rapid Interpretation of Electrocardiograms* (Tampa, Fla.: Cover Publishing Co., 1970).

Goldman, M. J.: *Principles of Clinical Electrocardiography* (7th ed.; Los Altos, Calif.: Lange Medical Series, 1970).

Hurst, J. W., and Myerburg, R. J.: *Introduction to Electrocardiography* (2d ed.; New York: McGraw-Hill Book Co., 1973).

Owens, S. G.: *Electrocardiography: A Programmed Text* (Boston: Little, Brown & Co., 1966).